Gluten Free Gestational Diabetes Cookbook

Jerry V. Hatcher

Table of Contents

Introduction

Bringing a new life into the world is a journey of unparalleled joy and anticipation. Yet, for many expecting mothers, the path to parenthood comes with unique challenges. This cookbook is crafted with love and understanding, designed to embrace the incredible journey of pregnancy, especially for those courageous women managing gestational diabetes while navigating the intricacies of a gluten-free lifestyle.

"Cooking for two" takes on a whole new meaning during pregnancy, and it is our sincere hope that this collection of recipes not only nourishes your body but also celebrates the profound beauty of this transformative time. Each dish is a testament to the belief that a health-conscious, gluten-free approach to nutrition can be both delicious and satisfying.

Within these pages, you'll find more than just recipes. This is a journey through flavors, a tapestry of ingredients woven together with care and consideration. We understand the challenges you face, the dietary restrictions that can sometimes feel like roadblocks, and the desire for meals that not only adhere to medical guidelines but also indulge the senses.

As you explore these recipes, you'll discover a diverse array of dishes – from hearty breakfasts that kickstart your day to comforting dinners meant to be shared with those you hold dear. Our hope is that this cookbook becomes a trusted companion, guiding you through the culinary aspects of your pregnancy with ease and joy.

This cookbook is a labor of love, born out of a deep commitment to supporting and nourishing mothers on their journey to motherhood. Here's to savoring each moment, to relishing the simple joys of a shared meal, and to the vibrant, delicious tapestry of a gluten-free, gestational diabetes-friendly kitchen.

With love and good health,

Jerry V. Hatcher

Overview of Gestational Diabetes

Gestational diabetes mellitus (GDM) is a form of diabetes that develops specifically during pregnancy. It is characterized by elevated blood sugar levels, and while it often resolves after childbirth, it requires careful management to ensure the health and well-being of both the mother and the developing baby.

Causes and Risk Factors:

Gestational diabetes occurs when the body is unable to produce sufficient insulin to meet the heightened demands during pregnancy. Various factors contribute to its development, including hormonal changes that affect insulin sensitivity. Women face an increased risk if they:

- Are overweight or obese before pregnancy.

- Have a family history of diabetes.

- Are over the age of 25.

- Belong to certain ethnic groups, such as African American, Hispanic, Native American, or Asian.

Effects on Pregnancy:

Untreated gestational diabetes can pose risks to both the mother and the baby. Complications may include:

1. Excessive Birth Weight: The baby may grow larger than average, increasing the risk of delivery complications.

2. Preterm Birth: Gestational diabetes can lead to an increased risk of preterm labor and delivery.

3. Low Blood Sugar in the Baby: After birth, the baby may experience low blood sugar levels due to the excess insulin produced in response to the mother's high blood sugar during pregnancy.

4. Type 2 Diabetes Risk: Mothers who have had gestational diabetes are at a higher risk of developing type 2 diabetes later in life.

Screening and Diagnosis:

Screening for gestational diabetes is a standard part of prenatal care. Typically, a glucose challenge test is conducted between 24 and 28 weeks of pregnancy. If the initial screening suggests elevated blood sugar levels, a follow-up glucose tolerance test may be performed to confirm the diagnosis.

Management and Treatment:

Managing gestational diabetes involves a combination of lifestyle changes, including:

1. Balanced Diet: A carefully planned diet that controls carbohydrate intake while ensuring proper nutrition for both mother and baby.

2. Regular Physical Activity: Moderate exercise helps regulate blood sugar levels.

3. Monitoring Blood Sugar Levels: Regular monitoring is essential to track blood sugar levels and ensure they stay within a healthy range.

In certain instances, the management of blood sugar levels may require the use of medication or insulin therapy. While gestational diabetes presents challenges, proper management significantly reduces associated risks. Through education, support, and a commitment to a healthy lifestyle, women can navigate gestational diabetes successfully, fostering a positive and nurturing environment for both mother and child.

Understanding Gluten-Free Living

Embarking on a gluten-free lifestyle involves more than just a dietary shift; it's a journey toward improved well-being and mindful choices. Whether prompted by health concerns, a celiac disease diagnosis, or a personal commitment to wellness, embracing gluten-free living requires knowledge, resilience, and creativity. Let's explore the essence of gluten-free living and the transformative impact it can have on your health.

1. What is Gluten?:

Gluten is a protein present in wheat, barley, rye, and related derivatives. While harmless for many, individuals with celiac disease or gluten sensitivity experience adverse reactions to gluten consumption, necessitating the elimination of gluten-containing foods from their diets.

2. The Gluten-Free Diet:

Adopting a gluten-free diet involves meticulous scrutiny of food labels and a conscious effort to select naturally gluten-free alternatives. Grains like rice, quinoa, and corn become staples, while gluten-free flours and products offer diverse possibilities for baking and cooking.

3. Health Benefits:

For those with gluten-related conditions, adhering to a gluten-free diet is paramount for alleviating symptoms and preventing long-term health complications. Beyond medical reasons, many individuals report increased energy levels, improved digestion, and enhanced overall well-being after transitioning to gluten-free living.

4. Gluten-Free Challenges:

Navigating a gluten-free lifestyle comes with its challenges. Social situations, dining out, and travel can pose dilemmas, requiring careful planning and communication. However, with a growing awareness of gluten intolerance, the availability of gluten-free options is expanding, making the journey more manageable.

5. Gluten-Free and Nutrient Balance:

While eliminating gluten is essential for some, maintaining a balanced and nutrient-rich diet is equally crucial. Incorporating a variety of naturally gluten-free whole foods ensures that the body receives the necessary vitamins, minerals, and fiber for optimal health.

6. Recipe Modification and Creativity:

Adapting traditional recipes to be gluten-free requires experimentation and an open mind. Fortunately, a plethora of gluten-free flours, alternative grains, and innovative cooking techniques empower individuals to savor familiar flavors without compromising on taste or texture.

7. Building a Supportive Community:

Embarking on a gluten-free journey is often more enjoyable when shared with a supportive community. Engaging with others who understand the challenges and triumphs creates a network of encouragement, recipe sharing, and shared experiences.

8. Embracing Gluten-Free Living:

Beyond the dietary aspect, gluten-free living encompasses a holistic approach to wellness. It encourages mindfulness about food choices, promotes self-care, and fosters a deeper connection with one's body. Embracing gluten-free living is not just a dietary adjustment but a lifestyle that prioritizes health, happiness, and a vibrant sense of well-being.

Importance of Nutrition During Pregnancy

Pregnancy is a transformative and awe-inspiring journey marked by the creation of new life. Central to the health and well-being of both the mother and the developing child is the role of nutrition. The choices made during these nine months profoundly impact the growth, development, and future health of the baby. Let's delve into the crucial importance of nutrition during pregnancy.

1. Nourishing Two Lives:

During pregnancy, the mother becomes the primary source of nourishment for her growing baby. Every nutrient, vitamin, and mineral consumed contributes to the formation of organs, tissues, and a foundation for a healthy life ahead.

2. Optimal Fetal Development:

Adequate nutrition is vital for the optimal development of the fetus. Essential nutrients such as folic acid, iron, calcium, and omega-3 fatty acids play pivotal roles in the formation of the neural tube, bones, and brain, fostering a healthy and resilient start to life.

3. Reducing the Risk of Birth Defects:

Proper nutrition significantly reduces the risk of birth defects and complications during pregnancy. For example, folic acid, particularly crucial in the early stages, helps prevent neural tube defects like spina bifida.

4. Healthy Weight Management:

Balanced nutrition supports healthy weight gain during pregnancy. Both insufficient and excessive weight gain can lead to complications, affecting not only the mother's health but also influencing the baby's growth and development.

5. Energy for the Journey:

The energy demands of pregnancy are substantial. Providing the body with a well-rounded, nutrient-dense diet ensures that the mother has the stamina and vitality needed for the physical and emotional demands of pregnancy, labor, and postpartum recovery.

6. Iron for Blood Health:

Iron plays a critical role in preventing anemia, a condition that can lead to fatigue and complications during pregnancy. Sufficient iron intake supports the increased blood volume needed to transport oxygen to the developing fetus.

7. Blood Sugar Regulation:

Maintaining stable blood sugar levels is essential to prevent gestational diabetes and ensure a healthy pregnancy. A diet rich in complex carbohydrates, fiber, and balanced meals helps regulate blood glucose levels.

8. Bone Health for Both:

Calcium is crucial for the development of the baby's bones and teeth. If the mother's calcium intake is inadequate, the body will draw from her own stores, potentially affecting her bone health.

9. Immune Support:

A body that is well-nourished is more effectively equipped to resist illnesses. Adequate intake of vitamins like C and D, as well as zinc, supports the immune system, benefitting both the mother and the developing baby.

10. Cognitive Development:

Omega-3 fatty acids, particularly DHA, are essential for the baby's cognitive development. Incorporating sources such as fatty fish and flaxseeds contributes to the formation of the baby's brain and nervous system.

In essence, nutrition during pregnancy is a cornerstone of maternal and fetal well-being. The choices made at the dining table resonate far beyond the immediate moment, shaping the health and vitality of generations to come.

Chapter 1: Breakfast Delights

1. Nutrient-Packed Berry Smoothie Bowl

A refreshing blend of mixed berries, Greek yogurt, and a touch of chia seeds. Packed with antioxidants, fiber, and protein, this smoothie bowl offers a delicious start to your day while helping stabilize blood sugar levels.

Ingredients:

- 1 cup mixed berries (strawberries, blueberries, raspberries)

- 1/2 cup Greek yogurt

- 1 tablespoon chia seeds

- 1/2 cup almond milk

- Ice cubes (optional)

Instructions:

1. In a blender, combine the mixed berries, Greek yogurt, chia seeds, and almond milk.

2. Blend until smooth, adding ice cubes if desired for a thicker consistency.

3. Pour the smoothie into a bowl.

4. Top with additional berries, a sprinkle of chia seeds, and a dollop of Greek yogurt.

Nutritional Information:

- Calories: ~250

- Protein: ~15g

- Carbohydrates: ~30g

- Fiber: ~8g

- Healthy fats: ~8g

2. Quinoa Breakfast Porridge with Almond Butter

A hearty quinoa porridge cooked in almond milk and topped with a spoonful of almond butter. Quinoa provides complex carbohydrates, fiber, and essential amino acids, offering a sustained energy release throughout the morning.

Ingredients:

- 1/2 cup quinoa, rinsed

- 1 cup almond milk

- 1 tablespoon almond butter

- 1 teaspoon honey or maple syrup

- Fresh fruit for topping (e.g., sliced banana or berries)

Instructions:

1. In a saucepan, combine quinoa and almond milk.

2. Bring to a boil, then reduce heat to simmer and cover. Cook until quinoa is tender and liquid is absorbed.

3. Stir in almond butter and sweeten with honey or maple syrup.

4. Top with fresh fruit before serving.

Nutritional Information:

- Calories: ~300

- Protein: ~10g

- Carbohydrates: ~40g

- Fiber: ~5g

- Healthy fats: ~10g

3. Egg White Vegetable Omelette

A light and fluffy omelette made with egg whites and loaded with colorful vegetables like bell peppers, spinach, and tomatoes. High in protein and low in fat, it's a satisfying and nutritious option for a gestational diabetes-friendly breakfast.

Ingredients:

- 3/4 cup egg whites

- 1/4 cup diced bell peppers (any color)

- 1/4 cup chopped spinach

- 1/4 cup diced tomatoes

- Salt and pepper to taste

- 1 teaspoon olive oil for cooking

 Instructions:

1. In a bowl, whisk together egg whites, bell peppers, spinach, and tomatoes.

2. Heat olive oil in a non-stick pan over medium heat.

3. Pour the egg mixture into the pan and cook until set.

4. Fold the omelette in half and serve.

Nutritional Information:

- Calories: ~150

- Protein: ~20g

- Carbohydrates: ~5g

- Fiber: ~2g

- Healthy fats: ~6g

4. Gluten-Free Pumpkin Pancakes

Fluffy pancakes made with gluten-free flour and infused with the warm flavors of pumpkin spice. Rich in fiber and low in added sugars, these pancakes are a delightful treat without compromising on nutritional balance.

Ingredients:

- 1 cup gluten-free pancake mix

- 1/2 cup pumpkin puree

- 1 teaspoon pumpkin spice

- 1 tablespoon maple syrup

- 1/2 cup almond milk

Instructions:

1. In a bowl, mix pancake mix, pumpkin puree, pumpkin spice, maple syrup, and almond milk until well combined.

2. Heat a griddle or non-stick pan over medium heat.

3. Pour 1/4 cup portions of batter onto the griddle.

4. Cook until bubbles form on the surface, then flip and cook until golden brown.

Nutritional Information:

- Calories: ~200

- Protein: ~4g

- Carbohydrates: ~35g

- Fiber: ~3g

- Healthy fats: ~5g

5. Chia Seed Pudding Parfait

Layers of chia seed pudding, fresh berries, and a dollop of Greek yogurt create a parfait that's not only visually appealing but also rich in omega-3 fatty acids, fiber, and probiotics.

Ingredients:

- 3 tablespoons chia seeds

- 1 cup almond milk

- 1/2 teaspoon vanilla extract

- 1 cup mixed berries

- 1/2 cup Greek yogurt

- Honey for drizzling

Instructions:

1. In a jar, mix chia seeds, almond milk, and vanilla extract. Stir well and refrigerate for at least 2 hours or overnight.

2. In a glass, layer chia pudding, mixed berries, and Greek yogurt.

3. Repeat the layers, finishing with a dollop of Greek yogurt.

4. Drizzle with honey before serving.

Nutritional Information:

- Calories: ~250

- Protein: ~10g

- Carbohydrates: ~30g

- Fiber: ~15g

- Healthy fats: ~10g

6. Vegetable and Feta Breakfast Casserole

A savory casserole featuring a medley of sautéed vegetables and feta cheese. High in fiber and protein, this make-ahead dish is perfect for busy mornings and provides a satisfying and balanced meal.

Ingredients:

- 1 cup chopped broccoli

- 1/2 cup diced bell peppers

- 1/2 cup cherry tomatoes, halved

- 4 eggs

- 1/2 cup crumbled feta cheese

- Salt and pepper to taste

Instructions:

1. Preheat the oven to 375°F (190°C).

2. In a bowl, whisk together eggs, salt, and pepper.

3. Grease a baking dish and spread chopped vegetables evenly.

4. Pour the whisked eggs over the vegetables.

5. Sprinkle crumbled feta on top.

6. Bake for 25-30 minutes or until the eggs are set.

Nutritional Information:

- Calories: ~250

- Protein: ~15g

- Carbohydrates: ~10g

- Fiber: ~3g

- Healthy fats: ~15g

7. Sweet Potato and Turkey Sausage Hash

A flavorful hash combining sweet potatoes, lean turkey sausage, and a mix of herbs. This dish is a low-carb, high-fiber option that's both hearty and gestational diabetes-friendly.

Ingredients:

- 1 cup diced sweet potatoes

- 1/2 cup lean turkey sausage, crumbled

- 1/4 cup diced onions

- 1/4 cup bell peppers, diced

- 1 tablespoon olive oil

- 1/2 teaspoon paprika

Instructions:

1. Heat olive oil in a skillet over medium heat.

2. Add sweet potatoes, turkey sausage, onions, and bell peppers.

3. Cook until sweet potatoes are tender and sausage is browned.

4. Sprinkle with paprika before serving.

Nutritional Information:

- Calories: ~300

- Protein: ~12g

- Carbohydrates: ~25g

- Fiber: ~5g

- Healthy fats: ~15g

8. Almond Flour Banana Muffins

Moist and tender banana muffins made with almond flour, providing a lower glycemic alternative to traditional muffins. These muffins are a delightful way to enjoy a sweet breakfast without spiking blood sugar levels.

Ingredients:

- 2 ripe bananas, mashed

- 2 cups almond flour

- 3 eggs

- 1/4 cup coconut oil, melted

- 1 teaspoon vanilla extract

- 1/2 teaspoon baking soda

Instructions:

1. Preheat the oven to 350°F (175°C).

2. In a bowl, combine mashed bananas, almond flour, eggs, melted coconut oil, vanilla extract, and baking soda.

3. Mix until well combined.

4. Spoon the batter into muffin cups and bake for 20-25 minutes.

Nutritional Information:

- Calories: ~200

- Protein: ~8g

- Carbohydrates: ~10g

- Fiber: ~3g

- Healthy fats: ~15g

9. Yogurt and Berry Parfait with Nuts

A parfait featuring layers of Greek yogurt, fresh berries, and a sprinkle of chopped nuts. This breakfast option offers a good balance of protein, healthy fats, and antioxidants to support overall health.

Ingredients:

- 1 cup Greek yogurt

- 1/2 cup mixed berries (strawberries, blueberries, raspberries)

- 2 tablespoons chopped nuts (almonds, walnuts)

- 1 tablespoon honey

Instructions:

1. In a glass, layer Greek yogurt, mixed berries, and chopped nuts.

2. Repeat the layers until the glass is filled.

3. Drizzle with honey before serving.

Nutritional Information:

- Calories: ~250

- Protein: ~15g

- Carbohydrates: ~20g

- Fiber: ~3g

- Healthy fats: ~12g

10. Oatmeal with Cinnamon and Walnuts

A classic bowl of oatmeal seasoned with cinnamon and topped with chopped walnuts. Oats are a slow-digesting whole grain, and combined with the heart-healthy fats from walnuts, this breakfast helps maintain steady blood sugar levels.

Ingredients:

- 1/2 cup old-fashioned oats

- 1 cup almond milk

- 1/2 teaspoon ground cinnamon

- 1/4 cup chopped walnuts

- 1 tablespoon maple syrup

 Instructions:

1. In a saucepan, combine oats and almond milk.

2. Cook over medium heat until the oats are tender.

3. Stir in ground cinnamon and top with chopped walnuts.

4. Drizzle with maple syrup before serving.

Nutritional Information:

- Calories: ~250

- Protein: ~8g

- Carbohydrates: ~30g

- Fiber: ~5g

- Healthy fats: ~10g

Each of these breakfast delights is crafted with the nutritional needs of gestational diabetes in mind, providing a mix of essential nutrients while keeping flavors delightful and satisfying.

Chapter 2: Lunchtime Favorites

1. Grilled Chicken and Avocado Salad

Tender grilled chicken breast slices atop a bed of fresh mixed greens, cherry tomatoes, and cucumber. Topped with creamy avocado slices and a light vinaigrette, this salad is a delicious and satisfying lunch option rich in lean protein and healthy fats.

Ingredients:

- 1 boneless, skinless chicken breast

- Mixed salad greens

- Cherry tomatoes, halved

- Cucumber, sliced

- Avocado, sliced

- Olive oil, for grilling

- Salt and pepper to taste

- Balsamic vinaigrette for dressing

Instructions:

1. Season the chicken breast with salt and pepper.

2. Grill the chicken until fully cooked.

3. In a large bowl, toss the mixed greens, cherry tomatoes, cucumber, and avocado slices.

4. Slice the grilled chicken and place it on top of the salad.

5. Drizzle with balsamic vinaigrette before serving.

Nutritional Information:

- Calories: ~350

- Protein: ~25g

- Carbohydrates: ~15g

- Fiber: ~8g

- Healthy fats: ~20g

2. Quinoa and Vegetable Stuffed Peppers

Colorful bell peppers stuffed with a hearty mixture of quinoa, black beans, corn, and diced vegetables. Baked to perfection, these stuffed peppers provide a nutrient-packed lunch with a balance of complex carbohydrates and fiber.

Ingredients:

- Bell peppers (any color), halved

- 1 cup cooked quinoa

- Black beans, drained and rinsed

- Corn kernels

- Diced tomatoes

- Onion, finely chopped

- Cumin, paprika, salt, and pepper to taste

- Shredded cheese for topping (optional)

Instructions:

1. Preheat the oven to 375°F (190°C).

2. In a bowl, mix cooked quinoa, black beans, corn, diced tomatoes, chopped onion, and seasonings.

3. Stuff the bell peppers with the quinoa mixture.

4. Place stuffed peppers in a baking dish and bake until peppers are tender.

5. Optionally, sprinkle with shredded cheese before serving.

Nutritional Information:

- Calories: ~300

- Protein: ~12g

- Carbohydrates: ~45g

- Fiber: ~8g

- Healthy fats: ~5g

3. Lentil Soup with Gluten-Free Bread

A comforting bowl of lentil soup featuring a medley of vegetables and aromatic spices. Served with a side of warm gluten-free bread, this lunch option is rich in fiber, protein, and essential nutrients to keep you satisfied throughout the day.

Ingredients:

- 1 cup dried lentils, rinsed

- Vegetable broth

- Carrots, celery, and onion, diced

- Garlic, minced

- Cumin, coriander, and turmeric to taste

- Salt and pepper to taste

- Gluten-free bread for serving

Instructions:

1. In a large pot, combine lentils, diced vegetables, garlic, and spices.

2. Add enough vegetable broth to cover the ingredients.

3. Simmer until lentils are tender.

4. Season with salt and pepper.

5. Serve with slices of gluten-free bread.

Nutritional Information:

- Calories: ~250

- Protein: ~15g

- Carbohydrates: ~40g

- Fiber: ~15g

- Healthy fats: ~2g

4. Zucchini Noodles with Pesto Sauce

Spiralized zucchini noodles tossed in a vibrant pesto sauce made with basil, pine nuts, and Parmesan cheese. This light and flavorful dish is a low-carb alternative to traditional pasta, providing a fresh and satisfying lunch.

Ingredients:

- Zucchini, spiralized

- Fresh basil leaves

- Pine nuts

- Parmesan cheese

- Garlic cloves

- Olive oil

- Salt and pepper to taste

Instructions:

1. In a food processor, blend basil, pine nuts, Parmesan, garlic, salt, and pepper.

2. While blending, gradually add olive oil until a smooth pesto sauce forms.

3. Toss spiralized zucchini with the pesto sauce.

4. Sauté in a pan until zucchini noodles are tender.

5. Serve warm.

Nutritional Information:

- Calories: ~200

- Protein: ~5g

- Carbohydrates: ~10g

- Fiber: ~4g

- Healthy fats: ~15g

5. Grilled Salmon and Quinoa Bowl

Grilled salmon fillet served over a bed of fluffy quinoa, accompanied by roasted vegetables and a drizzle of lemon-dill sauce. This bowl is a powerhouse of omega-3 fatty acids, lean protein, and whole grains for a nourishing and flavorful lunch.

Ingredients:

- Salmon fillet

- Quinoa, cooked

- Roasted vegetables (broccoli, bell peppers, etc.)

- Lemon-dill sauce (Greek yogurt, lemon juice, dill)

- Olive oil for grilling

- Salt and pepper to taste

Instructions:

1. Season the salmon with salt and pepper.

2. Grill the salmon until fully cooked.

3. In a bowl, assemble cooked quinoa, roasted vegetables, and grilled salmon.

4. Drizzle with lemon-dill sauce before serving.

 Nutritional Information:

- Calories: ~400

- Protein: ~30g

- Carbohydrates: ~30g

- Fiber: ~5g

- Healthy fats: ~18g

6. Turkey and Vegetable Stir-Fry

Lean ground turkey stir-fried with an assortment of colorful vegetables such as broccoli, bell peppers, and snap peas. Seasoned with ginger and garlic, this quick and nutritious stir-fry is served over cauliflower rice for a low-carb option.

Ingredients:

- Lean ground turkey

- Broccoli florets

- Bell peppers, sliced

- Snap peas

- Ginger and garlic, minced

- Low-sodium soy sauce

- Sesame oil

- Cauliflower rice for serving

Instructions:

1. In a wok or skillet, brown the ground turkey.

2. Add ginger, garlic, and vegetables; stir-fry until crisp-tender.

3. Add soy sauce and sesame oil for flavor.

4. Serve over cauliflower rice.

Nutritional Information:

- Calories: ~300

- Protein: ~20g

- Carbohydrates: ~15g

- Fiber: ~5g

- Healthy fats: ~10g

7. Eggplant Lasagna with Gluten-Free Pasta

Layers of thinly sliced eggplant, gluten-free lasagna noodles, and a savory tomato sauce, all baked to perfection. This gluten-free eggplant lasagna offers a satisfying and comforting lunch without compromising on flavor.

Ingredients:

- Eggplant, thinly sliced

- Gluten-free lasagna noodles

- Tomato sauce

- Ricotta cheese

- Mozzarella cheese, shredded

- Parmesan cheese, grated

- Italian seasoning

Instructions:

1. Preheat the oven to 375°F (190°C).

2. Layer sliced eggplant, gluten-free noodles, tomato sauce, and ricotta.

3. Repeat the layers, finishing with mozzarella and Parmesan.

4. Sprinkle with Italian seasoning.

5. Bake until bubbly and golden.

 Nutritional Information:

- Calories: ~350

- Protein: ~15g

- Carbohydrates: ~40g

- Fiber: ~8g

- Healthy fats: ~15g

8. Sweet Potato and Chickpea Curry

A flavorful curry made with sweet potatoes, chickpeas, and a blend of aromatic spices. Served over quinoa, this lunch option is rich in fiber, plant-based protein, and a variety of essential nutrients to support overall well-being.

Ingredients:

- Sweet potatoes, diced

- Chickpeas, drained and rinsed

- Coconut milk

- Curry powder, cumin, and turmeric

- Onion and garlic, minced

- Spinach leaves

- Quinoa for serving

Instructions:

1. In a pot, sauté onions and garlic until fragrant.

2. Add sweet potatoes, chickpeas, and spices.

3. Pour in coconut milk and simmer until sweet potatoes are tender.

4. Stir in spinach until wilted.

5. Serve over quinoa.

Nutritional Information:

- Calories: ~350

- Protein: ~12g

- Carbohydrates: ~50g

- Fiber: ~10g

- Healthy fats: ~10g

9. Mediterranean Quinoa Salad with Feta

A refreshing quinoa salad with cherry tomatoes, cucumber, Kalamata olives, and crumbled feta cheese. Tossed in a lemon-oregano dressing, this Mediterranean-inspired salad is a delightful and nutritious lunch option.

Ingredients:

- Quinoa, cooked

- Cherry tomatoes, halved

- Cucumber, diced

- Kalamata olives, sliced

- Feta cheese, crumbled

- Red onion, finely chopped

- Fresh oregano

- Olive oil and lemon juice dressing

Instructions:

1. In a large bowl, combine quinoa, tomatoes, cucumber, olives, feta, and red onion.

2. Toss with fresh oregano and dress with olive oil and lemon juice.

3. Mix well before serving.

Nutritional Information:

- Calories: ~300

- Protein: ~10g

- Carbohydrates: ~35g

- Fiber: ~6g

- Healthy fats: ~15g

10. Chicken and Vegetable Lettuce Wraps

Tender chicken strips sautéed with colorful bell peppers, carrots, and water chestnuts, seasoned with a flavorful ginger-soy sauce. Served in crisp lettuce leaves, these wraps offer a low-carb and satisfying lunch option.

Ingredients:

- Chicken breast, thinly sliced

- Bell peppers, julienned

- Carrots, julienned

- Water chestnuts, sliced

- Ginger and garlic, minced

- Low-sodium soy sauce

- Lettuce leaves for wrapping

Instructions:

1. In a skillet, sauté chicken, bell peppers, carrots, water chestnuts, ginger, and garlic.

2. Add soy sauce for flavor.

3. Spoon the mixture into lettuce leaves for wraps.

4. Serve with additional soy sauce if desired.

Nutritional Information:

- Calories: ~250

- Protein: ~18g

- Carbohydrates: ~15g

- Fiber: ~4g

- Healthy fats: ~8g

These lunchtime favorites are crafted with the nutritional needs of gestational diabetes in mind, providing a variety of flavors, textures, and nutrients to support a healthy and enjoyable lunch. Adjust portions and ingredients based on individual preferences and dietary requirements.

Chapter 3: Dinners for Two

1. Baked Lemon Herb Salmon

Tender salmon fillets marinated in a zesty lemon-herb mixture and baked to perfection. Served with a side of roasted vegetables, this dinner is rich in omega-3 fatty acids, lean protein, and fiber.

Ingredients:

- 2 salmon fillets

- 1 lemon, juiced and zested

- 2 tablespoons olive oil

- 2 cloves garlic, minced

- 1 teaspoon dried thyme

- Salt and pepper to taste

- Mixed vegetables (e.g., broccoli, cherry tomatoes)

Instructions:

1. Preheat the oven to 400°F (200°C).

2. In a bowl, whisk together lemon juice, lemon zest, olive oil, minced garlic, dried thyme, salt, and pepper.

3. Place salmon fillets on a baking sheet lined with parchment paper.

4. Pour the lemon herb mixture over the salmon.

5. Arrange mixed vegetables around the salmon.

6. Bake for 15-20 minutes or until the salmon is cooked through.

Nutritional Information (per serving):

- Calories: ~350

- Protein: ~30g

- Carbohydrates: ~10g

- Fiber: ~3g

- Healthy fats: ~20g

2. Turkey and Vegetable Skillet

Lean ground turkey cooked with a medley of colorful vegetables in a savory tomato sauce. This quick and flavorful skillet dinner is served over cauliflower rice for a low-carb option.

Ingredients:

- 1/2 lb lean ground turkey

- 1 bell pepper, diced

- 1 zucchini, sliced

- 1 cup cherry tomatoes, halved

- 1 can (14 oz) diced tomatoes

- 2 cloves garlic, minced

- Italian seasoning, salt, and pepper to taste

- Cauliflower rice for serving

Instructions:

1. In a skillet, brown ground turkey over medium heat.

2. Add diced bell pepper, sliced zucchini, halved cherry tomatoes, and minced garlic.

3. Pour in canned diced tomatoes and season with Italian seasoning, salt, and pepper.

4. Simmer until vegetables are tender.

5. Serve over cauliflower rice.

Nutritional Information (per serving):

- Calories: ~300

- Protein: ~20g

- Carbohydrates: ~15g

- Fiber: ~5g

- Healthy fats: ~15g

3. Eggplant and Chickpea Stew

A hearty stew featuring eggplant, chickpeas, and tomatoes simmered with aromatic spices. Served over quinoa, this dinner is a delicious combination of plant-based protein and complex carbohydrates.

Ingredients:

- 1 large eggplant, diced

- 1 can (15 oz) chickpeas, drained and rinsed

- 1 can (14 oz) diced tomatoes

- 1 onion, finely chopped

- 2 cloves garlic, minced

- 1 teaspoon cumin

- 1 teaspoon coriander

- 1 teaspoon turmeric

- Salt and pepper to taste

- Quinoa for serving

Instructions:

1. In a pot, sauté chopped onion and minced garlic until softened.

2. Add diced eggplant, chickpeas, diced tomatoes, and spices.

3. Season with salt and pepper.

4. Simmer until eggplant is tender.

5. Serve over cooked quinoa.

Nutritional Information (per serving):

- Calories: ~350

- Protein: ~15g

- Carbohydrates: ~50g

- Fiber: ~15g

- Healthy fats: ~8g

4. Cauliflower Crust Pizza

A homemade cauliflower crust topped with tomato sauce, lean protein (chicken or turkey), and a variety of vegetables. This pizza is a low-carb alternative that doesn't compromise on taste.

Ingredients:

- 1 medium-sized cauliflower

- 1 egg

- 1/2 cup grated Parmesan cheese

- 1/2 teaspoon dried oregano

- 1/2 teaspoon garlic powder

- Tomato sauce, lean protein (chicken or turkey), vegetables

- Mozzarella cheese for topping

Instructions:

1. Preheat the oven to 425°F (220°C).

2. Grate the cauliflower and microwave for 5 minutes.

3. Allow the cauliflower to cool, then mix with egg, Parmesan, oregano, and garlic powder.

4. Form the mixture into a crust on a baking sheet and bake for 15-20 minutes.

5. Remove from the oven, add tomato sauce, lean protein, vegetables, and top with mozzarella.

6. Bake until the cheese is melted and bubbly.

Nutritional Information (per serving):

- Calories: ~250

- Protein: ~15g

- Carbohydrates: ~20g

- Fiber: ~8g

- Healthy fats: ~12g

5. Stir-Fried Shrimp with Broccoli

Succulent shrimp stir-fried with crisp broccoli and bell peppers in a light ginger-soy sauce. Served over a bed of cauliflower rice, this dinner is a tasty and low-carb option.

Ingredients:

- 1/2 lb shrimp, peeled and deveined

- 2 cups broccoli florets

- 1 bell pepper, sliced

- 2 cloves garlic, minced

- 2 tablespoons low-sodium soy sauce

- 1 tablespoon sesame oil

- 1 teaspoon ginger, grated

- Cauliflower rice for serving

Instructions:

1. In a wok or skillet, sauté shrimp until pink and opaque. Remove from the pan.

2. Stir-fry broccoli and bell pepper until crisp-tender.

3. Add minced garlic and grated ginger.

4. Return shrimp to the pan, add soy sauce, and drizzle with sesame oil.

5. Stir-fry until well combined.

6. Serve over cauliflower rice.

Nutritional Information (per serving):

- Calories: ~280

- Protein: ~25g

- Carbohydrates: ~15g

- Fiber: ~6g

- Healthy fats: ~12g

6. Grilled Chicken and Vegetable Kebabs

Marinated chicken breast and colorful vegetables threaded onto skewers and grilled to perfection. Served with a side of quinoa, these kebabs offer a balanced combination of protein and fiber.

Ingredients:

- 2 boneless, skinless chicken breasts, cut into cubes

- Bell peppers, cherry tomatoes, and red onion, cut into chunks

- Olive oil

- Lemon juice

- Garlic powder, paprika, salt, and pepper to taste

- Quinoa for serving

Instructions:

1. In a bowl, combine chicken cubes, vegetables, olive oil, lemon juice, and seasonings.

2. Thread the chicken and vegetables onto skewers.

3. Grill until chicken is cooked through and vegetables are tender.

4. Serve over a bed of quinoa.

 Nutritional Information (per serving):

- Calories: ~350

- Protein: ~30g

- Carbohydrates: ~25g

- Fiber: ~5g

- Healthy fats: ~15g

7. Spaghetti Squash with Turkey Bolognese

Roasted spaghetti squash strands tossed with a flavorful turkey Bolognese sauce. This dinner is a satisfying, low-carb alternative to traditional pasta dishes.

Ingredients:

- 1 medium-sized spaghetti squash

- 1/2 lb lean ground turkey

- 1 can (14 oz) crushed tomatoes

- Garlic, minced

- Italian seasoning, salt, and pepper to taste

- Fresh basil for garnish

Instructions:

1. Preheat the oven to 400°F (200°C).

2. Cut the spaghetti squash in half and remove the seeds.

3. Roast the squash in the oven until the flesh is tender.

4. In a skillet, brown ground turkey and add minced garlic.

5. Pour in crushed tomatoes and season with Italian seasoning, salt, and pepper.

6. Scrape the spaghetti squash with a fork to create "noodles."

7. Top with turkey Bolognese and garnish with fresh basil.

Nutritional Information (per serving):

- Calories: ~320

- Protein: ~20g

- Carbohydrates: ~30g

- Fiber: ~8g

- Healthy fats: ~15g

8. Salmon and Asparagus Foil Packets

Salmon fillets and fresh asparagus spears seasoned with herbs, garlic, and lemon, wrapped in foil and baked. This easy and delicious dinner is a source of heart-healthy fats and nutrients.

Ingredients:

- 2 salmon fillets

- Fresh asparagus spears

- Lemon slices

- Olive oil

- Garlic, minced

- Dill, salt, and pepper to taste

- Quinoa for serving

Instructions:

1. Preheat the oven to 400°F (200°C).

2. Place each salmon fillet on a piece of foil.

3. Arrange asparagus spears around the salmon.

4. Drizzle with olive oil and sprinkle with minced garlic, dill, salt, and pepper.

5. Seal the foil packets and bake for 15-20 minutes.

6. Serve over a bed of quinoa.

Nutritional Information (per serving):

- Calories: ~380

- Protein: ~30g

- Carbohydrates: ~20g

- Fiber: ~5g

- Healthy fats: ~20g

9. Mushroom and Spinach Stuffed Chicken Breast

Chicken breasts filled with a savory mixture of mushrooms, spinach, and feta cheese. Baked to perfection, this dish is a flavorful and protein-rich option for a healthy dinner for two.

Ingredients:

- 2 boneless, skinless chicken breasts

- Mushrooms, chopped

- Fresh spinach leaves

- Feta cheese, crumbled

- Olive oil

- Garlic powder, paprika, salt, and pepper to taste

- Quinoa for serving

Instructions:

1. Preheat the oven to 375°F (190°C).

2. Butterfly the chicken breasts and pound them thin.

3. Sauté mushrooms in olive oil until tender.

4. Layer spinach, sautéed mushrooms, and crumbled feta on each chicken breast.

5. Fold the chicken and secure with toothpicks.

6. Season with garlic powder, paprika, salt, and pepper.

7. Bake until chicken is cooked through.

8. Serve over a bed of quinoa.

Nutritional Information (per serving):

- Calories: ~340

- Protein: ~30g

- Carbohydrates: ~20g

- Fiber: ~4g

- Healthy fats: ~15g

10. Vegetarian Zucchini Boat Casserole

Zucchini boats filled with a hearty mixture of quinoa, black beans, corn, and diced tomatoes. Baked until golden, this vegetarian casserole is a nutritious and satisfying option for two.

Ingredients:

- 2 large zucchinis, halved and scooped

- 1 cup cooked quinoa

- 1 can (15 oz) black beans, drained and rinsed

- 1 cup corn kernels

- 1 can (14 oz) diced tomatoes

- 1 teaspoon cumin, chili powder, and garlic powder

- Shredded cheddar cheese for topping

Instructions:

1. Preheat the oven to 375°F (190°C).

2. In a bowl, mix cooked quinoa, black beans, corn, diced tomatoes, and spices.

3. Fill each zucchini boat with the quinoa mixture.

4. Top with shredded cheddar cheese.

5. Bake until zucchini is tender and cheese is melted.

Nutritional Information (per serving):

- Calories: ~320

- Protein: ~15g

- Carbohydrates: ~50g

- Fiber: ~12g

- Healthy fats: ~8g

These dinner recipes for two are crafted with the nutritional needs of gestational diabetes in mind, providing a variety of flavors and nutrients to enjoy while managing blood sugar levels.

Chapter 4: Snack Attack

1. Greek Yogurt and Berry Parfait

A delightful snack featuring layers of Greek yogurt, fresh berries (such as strawberries, blueberries, and raspberries), and a sprinkle of chopped nuts. This parfait is rich in protein, antioxidants, and healthy fats.

Ingredients:

- 1 cup Greek yogurt

- Mixed berries (strawberries, blueberries, raspberries)

- Chopped nuts (almonds, walnuts)

Instructions:

1. In a glass or bowl, layer Greek yogurt with fresh berries.

2. Top with a sprinkle of chopped nuts.

3. Repeat the layers.

4. Enjoy this protein-packed and antioxidant-rich parfait!

Nutritional Information (per serving):

- Calories: ~200

- Protein: ~15g

- Carbohydrates: ~20g

- Fiber: ~4g

- Healthy fats: ~8g

2. Cucumber and Hummus Bites

Sliced cucumbers topped with a dollop of hummus. This snack provides a refreshing crunch, fiber from the cucumber, and the satisfying protein and healthy fats from hummus.

Ingredients:

- Cucumber, sliced

- Hummus

Instructions:

1. Slice cucumbers into rounds.

2. Top each cucumber slice with a small dollop of hummus.

3. Arrange on a plate and enjoy this refreshing and satisfying snack!

Nutritional Information (per serving):

- Calories: ~100

- Protein: ~3g

- Carbohydrates: ~10g

- Fiber: ~3g

- Healthy fats: ~6g

3. Cheese and Whole Grain Crackers

A combination of sliced cheese (such as cheddar or mozzarella) paired with whole grain crackers. This snack offers a balance of protein, whole grains, and calcium.

Ingredients:

- Cheese slices (cheddar, mozzarella)

- Whole grain crackers

Instructions:

1. Slice cheese into portions.

2. Pair each cheese slice with whole grain crackers.

3. Enjoy this simple and balanced snack!

Nutritional Information (per serving):

- Calories: ~150

- Protein: ~8g

- Carbohydrates: ~10g

- Fiber: ~2g

- Healthy fats: ~9g

4. Almond Butter and Banana Slices

Banana slices smeared with almond butter. This snack is a tasty and energizing option, providing potassium from bananas and healthy fats from almond butter.

Ingredients:

- Banana, sliced

- Almond butter

Instructions:

1. Slice bananas into rounds.

2. Spread almond butter on each banana slice.

3. Arrange on a plate and savor the combination of sweetness and creaminess!

Nutritional Information (per serving):

- Calories: ~180

- Protein: ~4g

- Carbohydrates: ~20g

- Fiber: ~4g

- Healthy fats: ~10g

5. Vegetable Sticks with Tzatziki

Crisp vegetable sticks (carrots, bell peppers, and cucumber) served with a side of homemade tzatziki. This snack is low in carbohydrates and high in fiber and vitamins.

Ingredients:

- Carrot sticks

- Bell pepper strips

- Cucumber sticks

- Tzatziki for dipping

Instructions:

1. Cut vegetables into stick shapes.

2. Serve with a side of tzatziki for a refreshing and low-carb snack.

Nutritional Information (per serving):

- Calories: ~80

- Protein: ~2g

- Carbohydrates: ~10g

- Fiber: ~3g

- Healthy fats: ~4g

6. Hard-Boiled Eggs with Avocado

Sliced hard-boiled eggs topped with creamy avocado slices. This snack is rich in protein, healthy fats, and essential nutrients.

Ingredients:

- Hard-boiled eggs

- Avocado, sliced

- Salt and pepper to taste

Instructions:

1. Slice hard-boiled eggs in half.

2. Top each half with a slice of avocado.

3. Sprinkle with salt and pepper.

4. Enjoy this protein-rich and satisfying snack!

Nutritional Information (per serving):

- Calories: ~200

- Protein: ~12g

- Carbohydrates: ~7g

- Fiber: ~5g

- Healthy fats: ~14g

7. Trail Mix with Nuts and Seeds

A mix of nuts (such as almonds and walnuts) and seeds (pumpkin seeds and sunflower seeds), with a sprinkle of dried berries. This snack provides a satisfying crunch, protein, and omega-3 fatty acids.

Ingredients:

- Almonds

- Walnuts

- Pumpkin seeds

- Sunflower seeds

- Dried berries (cranberries, blueberries)

Instructions:

1. Mix almonds, walnuts, pumpkin seeds, sunflower seeds, and dried berries in a bowl.

2. Portion into snack-sized servings.

3. Enjoy this nutrient-dense and satisfying trail mix!

Nutritional Information (per serving):

- Calories: ~250

- Protein: ~8g

- Carbohydrates: ~15g

- Fiber: ~5g

- Healthy fats: ~18g

8. Cherry Tomato and Mozzarella Skewers

Skewers alternating cherry tomatoes and fresh mozzarella balls, drizzled with balsamic glaze. This snack is a flavorful and portion-controlled option.

Ingredients:

- Cherry tomatoes

- Fresh mozzarella balls

- Balsamic glaze

Instructions:

1. Thread cherry tomatoes and fresh mozzarella balls onto skewers.

2. Drizzle with balsamic glaze.

3. Serve these flavorful and portion-controlled skewers!

Nutritional Information (per serving):

- Calories: ~120

- Protein: ~6g

- Carbohydrates: ~5g

- Fiber: ~1g

- Healthy fats: ~8g

9. Apple Slices with Peanut Butter

Crisp apple slices paired with natural peanut butter. This snack combines the sweetness of apples with the protein and healthy fats from peanut butter.

Ingredients:

- Apple, sliced

- Natural peanut butter

Instructions:

1. Slice apples into wedges.

2. Spread natural peanut butter on each wedge.

3. Enjoy the sweet and savory combination of flavors!

Nutritional Information (per serving):

- Calories: ~180

- Protein: ~4g

- Carbohydrates: ~20g

- Fiber: ~5g

- Healthy fats: ~10g

10. Yogurt-Covered Almonds

Almonds coated in a thin layer of yogurt and chilled until set. This snack provides a satisfying combination of protein, healthy fats, and a touch of sweetness.

Ingredients:

- Almonds

- Greek yogurt

- Honey (optional)

Instructions:

1. Dip almonds in Greek yogurt.

2. Place on a tray and freeze until yogurt is set.

3. Optionally, drizzle with honey for sweetness.

4. Enjoy these crunchy and satisfying yogurt-covered almonds!

Nutritional Information (per serving):

- Calories: ~180

- Protein: ~6g

- Carbohydrates: ~10g

- Fiber: ~3g

- Healthy fats: ~14g

Chapter 5: Sweet Treats

1. Berry and Greek Yogurt Popsicles

Refreshing popsicles made with a blend of mixed berries and Greek yogurt. These frozen treats are low in added sugars and high in antioxidants and probiotics.

Ingredients:

- 1 cup mixed berries (strawberries, blueberries, raspberries)

- 1 cup Greek yogurt

- 1-2 tablespoons honey or sweetener of choice

Instructions:

1. Blend mixed berries with Greek yogurt and sweetener until smooth.

2. Pour the mixture into popsicle molds.

3. Freeze until solid.

4. Enjoy these refreshing and protein-packed popsicles!

Nutritional Information (per serving):

- Calories: ~80

- Protein: ~5g

- Carbohydrates: ~15g

- Fiber: ~2g

- Healthy fats: ~1g

2. Dark Chocolate-Dipped Strawberries

Juicy strawberries dipped in dark chocolate. This sweet treat offers a satisfying combination of antioxidants from dark chocolate and essential vitamins from strawberries.

Ingredients:

- Fresh strawberries

- Dark chocolate (70% cocoa or higher)

 Instructions:

1. Melt dark chocolate in a heatproof bowl.

2. Dip each strawberry into the melted chocolate.

3. Place on parchment paper and let it cool.

4. Indulge in these sweet and antioxidant-rich treats!

Nutritional Information (per serving):

- Calories: ~50

- Protein: ~1g

- Carbohydrates: ~8g

- Fiber: ~2g

- Healthy fats: ~3g

3. Chia Seed Pudding with Almond Milk

Creamy chia seed pudding made with almond milk, sweetened with a touch of natural sweeteners like stevia or monk fruit. This pudding is high in fiber and omega-3 fatty acids.

Ingredients:

- 3 tablespoons chia seeds

- 1 cup unsweetened almond milk

- 1-2 tablespoons sweetener of choice (stevia, monk fruit)

- 1/2 teaspoon vanilla extract

Instructions:

1. Mix chia seeds, almond milk, sweetener, and vanilla extract in a bowl.

2. Refrigerate for at least 2 hours or overnight.

3. Stir well before serving.

4. Enjoy this fiber-rich and omega-3 packed pudding!

Nutritional Information (per serving):

- Calories: ~120

- Protein: ~4g

- Carbohydrates: ~12g

- Fiber: ~8g

- Healthy fats: ~7g

4. Baked Apple with Cinnamon

Sliced apples baked with a sprinkle of cinnamon. This warm and comforting treat is naturally sweetened with the caramelized sugars from the baked apples.

Ingredients:

- Apple, sliced

- Cinnamon

- Optional: A sprinkle of nutmeg or a drizzle of honey

Instructions:

1. Preheat the oven to 375°F (190°C).

2. Place apple slices on a baking sheet.

3. Sprinkle with cinnamon (and nutmeg or honey if desired).

4. Bake until apples are tender.

5. Savor the warm and naturally sweetened baked apples!

Nutritional Information (per serving):

- Calories: ~60

- Protein: ~0g

- Carbohydrates: ~15g

- Fiber: ~3g

- Healthy fats: ~0g

5. Frozen Banana Bites

Banana slices dipped in a thin layer of yogurt, then frozen. These bite-sized treats offer natural sweetness, potassium, and a satisfying crunch.

Ingredients:

- Bananas, sliced

- Greek yogurt

- Optional: Unsweetened shredded coconut or chopped nuts

 Instructions:

1. Dip banana slices in Greek yogurt.

2. Place on a tray lined with parchment paper.

3. Optional: Sprinkle with shredded coconut or chopped nuts.

4. Freeze until solid.

5. Enjoy these frozen, creamy, and naturally sweet banana bites!

 Nutritional Information (per serving):

- Calories: ~70

- Protein: ~2g

- Carbohydrates: ~15g

- Fiber: ~1g

- Healthy fats: ~1g

6. Almond Flour Blueberry Muffins

Moist and fluffy blueberry muffins made with almond flour, sweetened with a sugar substitute like erythritol or stevia. These muffins are lower in carbohydrates and higher in healthy fats.

Ingredients:

- 1 cup almond flour

- 1/4 cup coconut flour

- 1/2 teaspoon baking powder

- Pinch of salt

- 1/4 cup melted coconut oil

- 1/4 cup unsweetened almond milk

- 2 eggs

- 1/4 cup sugar substitute (erythritol or stevia)

- 1 teaspoon vanilla extract

- 1/2 cup fresh or frozen blueberries

Instructions:

1. Preheat the oven to 350°F (175°C).

2. In a bowl, whisk together almond flour, coconut flour, baking powder, and salt.

3. In another bowl, mix melted coconut oil, almond milk, eggs, sugar substitute, and vanilla extract.

4. Combine wet and dry ingredients, then fold in blueberries.

5. Spoon the batter into muffin cups and bake for 20-25 minutes.

6. Allow to cool before enjoying these low-carb blueberry muffins!

Nutritional Information (per serving):

- Calories: ~150

- Protein: ~5g

- Carbohydrates: ~10g

- Fiber: ~3g

- Healthy fats: ~10g

7. Avocado Chocolate Mousse

Silky chocolate mousse made with ripe avocados, cocoa powder, and a natural sweetener. This rich and indulgent treat is packed with healthy fats and antioxidants.

Ingredients:

- 2 ripe avocados

- 1/4 cup unsweetened cocoa powder

- 1/4 cup almond milk

- 1/4 cup sugar substitute (stevia or monk fruit)

- 1 teaspoon vanilla extract

- Pinch of salt

Instructions:

1. Blend avocados, cocoa powder, almond milk, sugar substitute, vanilla extract, and salt until smooth.

2. Chill in the refrigerator.

3. Spoon into serving dishes.

4. Indulge in this creamy and rich chocolate mousse!

Nutritional Information (per serving):

- Calories: ~150

- Protein: ~3g

- Carbohydrates: ~10g

- Fiber: ~6g

- Healthy fats: ~12g

8. Coconut and Almond Energy Balls

No-bake energy balls made with shredded coconut, almonds, and a hint of vanilla. These bites provide a quick energy boost without a spike in blood sugar levels.

Ingredients:

- 1 cup shredded coconut

- 1/2 cup almond flour

- 1/4 cup almond butter

- 2 tablespoons honey or sweetener of choice

- 1 teaspoon vanilla extract

- Pinch of salt

Instructions:

1. In a bowl, mix shredded coconut, almond flour, almond butter, honey, vanilla extract, and salt.

2. Form into small balls and refrigerate until firm.

3. Enjoy these no-bake energy balls for a quick and nutritious snack!

Nutritional Information (per serving):

- Calories: ~100

- Protein: ~2g

- Carbohydrates: ~6g

- Fiber: ~2g

- Healthy fats: ~8g

9. Cinnamon Baked Pears

Pears sliced and baked with a sprinkle of cinnamon. This warm dessert is a simple and nutritious way to satisfy sweet cravings.

Ingredients:

- Pears, halved and cored

- Cinnamon

- Optional: A sprinkle of nutmeg or a drizzle of honey

 Instructions:

1. Preheat the oven to 375°F (190°C).

2. Place pear halves on a baking sheet.

3. Sprinkle with cinnamon (and nutmeg or honey if desired).

4. Bake until pears are tender.

5. Enjoy these warm and naturally sweetened baked pears!

 Nutritional Information (per serving):

- Calories: ~80

- Protein: ~0g

- Carbohydrates: ~20g

- Fiber: ~4g

- Healthy fats: ~0g

10. Pumpkin Spice Chia Pudding

Chia pudding infused with pumpkin spice flavors, made with unsweetened almond milk. This seasonal treat is rich in fiber, vitamins, and minerals.

Ingredients:

- 3 tablespoons chia seeds

- 1 cup unsweetened almond milk

- 1/4 cup canned pumpkin puree

- 1-2 tablespoons sweetener of choice (stevia, monk fruit)

- 1/2 teaspoon pumpkin spice

 Instructions:

1. Mix chia seeds, almond milk, pumpkin puree, sweetener, and pumpkin spice in a bowl.

2. Refrigerate for at least 2 hours or overnight.

3. Stir well before serving.

4. Enjoy this seasonal and fiber-rich pumpkin spice chia pudding!

Nutritional Information (per serving):

- Calories: ~120

- Protein: ~3g

- Carbohydrates: ~12g

- Fiber: ~8g

- Healthy fats: ~7g

Chapter 6: Sides and Extras

1. Quinoa and Vegetable Stuffed Bell Peppers

Bell peppers filled with a mixture of cooked quinoa, assorted vegetables, and lean protein. This side dish is rich in fiber, vitamins, and minerals.

Ingredients:

- Bell peppers, halved and seeds removed

- Cooked quinoa

- Mixed vegetables (zucchini, cherry tomatoes, onions)

- Lean protein (chicken or turkey)

- Olive oil, garlic, salt, and pepper

Instructions:

1. Preheat the oven to 375°F (190°C).

2. In a bowl, mix cooked quinoa, diced vegetables, lean protein, olive oil, garlic, salt, and pepper.

3. Stuff the bell peppers with the quinoa mixture.

4. Bake until peppers are tender.

5. Serve these nutrient-packed stuffed bell peppers as a delicious side dish!

Nutritional Information (per serving):

- Calories: ~180

- Protein: ~15g

- Carbohydrates: ~20g

- Fiber: ~4g

- Healthy fats: ~6g

2. Garlic Roasted Brussels Sprouts

Brussels sprouts roasted with garlic, olive oil, and a touch of sea salt. This flavorful side is low in carbohydrates and high in fiber.

Ingredients:

- Brussels sprouts, halved

- Olive oil

- Minced garlic

- Sea salt and black pepper

Instructions:

1. Preheat the oven to 400°F (200°C).

2. Toss Brussels sprouts with olive oil, minced garlic, sea salt, and black pepper.

3. Roast until Brussels sprouts are golden brown.

4. Enjoy these flavorful garlic roasted Brussels sprouts as a low-carb side!

Nutritional Information (per serving):

- Calories: ~90

- Protein: ~4g

- Carbohydrates: ~10g

- Fiber: ~4g

- Healthy fats: ~5g

3. Cauliflower Mash

Creamy mashed cauliflower seasoned with garlic and herbs. This low-carb alternative to mashed potatoes is a tasty and nutritious side.

Ingredients:

- Cauliflower florets

- Garlic, minced

- Greek yogurt or cream cheese

- Salt and pepper

- Chopped chives for garnish

Instructions:

1. Steam or boil cauliflower until tender.

2. Mash cauliflower with minced garlic, Greek yogurt or cream cheese, salt, and pepper.

3. Garnish with chopped chives.

4. Enjoy this creamy and low-carb alternative to mashed potatoes!

Nutritional Information (per serving):

- Calories: ~70

- Protein: ~3g

- Carbohydrates: ~8g

- Fiber: ~4g

- Healthy fats: ~3g

4. Spinach and Feta Stuffed Mushrooms

Mushrooms stuffed with a mixture of spinach, feta cheese, and herbs. These bite-sized delights are packed with iron and protein.

Ingredients:

- Large mushrooms, stems removed

- Fresh spinach, chopped

- Feta cheese, crumbled

- Garlic, minced

- Olive oil, salt, and pepper

Instructions:

1. Preheat the oven to 375°F (190°C).

2. In a pan, sauté spinach and minced garlic in olive oil until wilted.

3. Mix spinach with crumbled feta, salt, and pepper.

4. Stuff mushrooms with the spinach and feta mixture.

5. Bake until mushrooms are tender.

6. Enjoy these bite-sized stuffed mushrooms as a savory side!

Nutritional Information (per serving):

- Calories: ~80

- Protein: ~5g

- Carbohydrates: ~4g

- Fiber: ~2g

- Healthy fats: ~6g

5. Zucchini Noodles with Pesto

Zucchini noodles tossed in homemade pesto made with basil, garlic, pine nuts, and Parmesan. This low-carb alternative to pasta is a fresh and flavorful side.

Ingredients:

- Zucchini, spiralized into noodles

- Fresh basil, garlic, pine nuts, and Parmesan for pesto

- Cherry tomatoes, halved

Instructions:

1. Spiralize zucchini into noodles.

2. In a blender, combine fresh basil, garlic, pine nuts, and Parmesan to make pesto.

3. Toss zucchini noodles with pesto and cherry tomatoes.

4. Serve this low-carb and flavorful zucchini noodle dish as a side!

Nutritional Information (per serving):

- Calories: ~120

- Protein: ~4g

- Carbohydrates: ~8g

- Fiber: ~3g

- Healthy fats: ~9g

6. Roasted Sweet Potato Wedges

Sweet potato wedges roasted with a drizzle of olive oil and a sprinkle of cinnamon. This side dish provides complex carbohydrates and is rich in beta-carotene.

Ingredients:

- Sweet potatoes, cut into wedges

- Olive oil

- Cinnamon

- Sea salt

 Instructions:

1. Preheat the oven to 400°F (200°C).

2. Toss sweet potato wedges with olive oil, cinnamon, and sea salt.

3. Roast until the edges are golden brown.

4. Enjoy these flavorful and nutrient-rich sweet potato wedges as a satisfying side!

 Nutritional Information (per serving):

- Calories: ~100

- Protein: ~2g

- Carbohydrates: ~20g

- Fiber: ~3g

- Healthy fats: ~2g

7. Broccoli and Cauliflower Gratin

Broccoli and cauliflower florets baked in a cheesy gratin with a hint of nutmeg. This side is a delicious way to incorporate cruciferous vegetables into your meal.

Ingredients:

- Broccoli and cauliflower florets

- Grated Parmesan cheese

- Nutmeg

- Greek yogurt or cream cheese

Instructions:

1. Preheat the oven to 375°F (190°C).

2. Steam or boil broccoli and cauliflower until tender.

3. Mix with Greek yogurt or cream cheese, grated Parmesan, and a pinch of nutmeg.

4. Bake until the top is golden and bubbly.

5. Savor this cheesy and nutritious gratin as a tasty side!

Nutritional Information (per serving):

- Calories: ~120

- Protein: ~6g

- Carbohydrates: ~10g

- Fiber: ~4g

- Healthy fats: ~6g

8. Cucumber and Tomato Salad with Balsamic Vinaigrette

Refreshing salad with cucumber slices, cherry tomatoes, and a light balsamic vinaigrette. This side is low in carbohydrates and high in hydration.

Ingredients:

- Cucumber, sliced

- Cherry tomatoes, halved

- Red onion, thinly sliced

- Balsamic vinaigrette (olive oil, balsamic vinegar, Dijon mustard, garlic, salt, and pepper)

Instructions:

1. In a bowl, combine cucumber slices, cherry tomatoes, and sliced red onion.

2. Drizzle with balsamic vinaigrette and toss.

3. Refrigerate before serving.

4. Enjoy this refreshing and hydrating cucumber and tomato salad!

Nutritional Information (per serving):

- Calories: ~60

- Protein: ~1g

- Carbohydrates: ~8g

- Fiber: ~2g

- Healthy fats: ~4g

9. Asparagus with Lemon and Parmesan

Asparagus spears roasted with fresh lemon juice and grated Parmesan. This side dish is a simple and nutritious way to enjoy seasonal vegetables.

Ingredients:

- Fresh asparagus spears

- Lemon zest

- Grated Parmesan cheese

- Olive oil

- Salt and pepper

Instructions:

1. Preheat the oven to 400°F (200°C).

2. Arrange asparagus on a baking sheet.

3. Drizzle with olive oil, lemon zest, grated Parmesan, salt, and pepper.

4. Roast until asparagus is tender.

5. Enjoy this zesty and nutritious asparagus side!

Nutritional Information (per serving):

- Calories: ~70

- Protein: ~4g

- Carbohydrates: ~6g

- Fiber: ~3g

- Healthy fats: ~5g

10. Mashed Avocado with Tomato Salsa

Ripe avocado mashed and topped with a zesty tomato salsa. This side provides healthy fats, vitamins, and a burst of flavor.

Ingredients:

- Ripe avocados, mashed

- Tomatoes, diced

- Red onion, finely chopped

- Cilantro, chopped

- Lime juice

- Salt and pepper

Instructions:

1. Mash ripe avocados in a bowl.

2. In another bowl, mix diced tomatoes, chopped red onion, cilantro, lime juice, salt, and pepper to make salsa.

3. Top mashed avocados with tomato salsa.

4. Enjoy this simple and flavorful mashed avocado with tomato salsa!

Nutritional Information (per serving):

- Calories: ~120

- Protein: ~2g

- Carbohydrates: ~8g

- Fiber: ~5g

- Healthy fats: ~10g

Chapter 7: Tips for Managing Gestational Diabetes

Understanding Blood Sugar Levels

Blood sugar levels play a crucial role in the health and well-being of both the mother and the baby during pregnancy, particularly when managing gestational diabetes. Here's a breakdown to help you better comprehend this essential aspect of health:

What Are Blood Sugar Levels?

Blood sugar, or glucose, is a form of sugar that circulates in our bloodstream and serves as the primary source of energy for our cells. It comes from the food we eat, especially carbohydrates. During pregnancy, hormonal changes can affect how the body processes and uses glucose.

Normal Blood Sugar Levels During Pregnancy

Maintaining stable blood sugar levels is pivotal to managing gestational diabetes. Healthcare providers typically establish target blood sugar ranges for pregnant individuals. This includes fasting levels (measured before meals) and post-meal levels (measured after meals). Uncontrolled blood sugar levels during pregnancy can have adverse effects on the health of the baby, making monitoring and regulation critical.

Monitoring Blood Sugar Levels

Regular monitoring of blood sugar levels is a cornerstone of gestational diabetes management. Healthcare providers often recommend the use of glucose meters, allowing pregnant individuals to measure their blood sugar levels at various times throughout the day. Keeping a blood sugar log helps identify patterns and trends, aiding in the development of an effective management plan.

Factors Affecting Blood Sugar Levels

Several factors can influence blood sugar levels, and understanding them is key to effective management. Diet, physical activity, stress, and hormonal changes can all contribute to fluctuations. Recognizing and addressing these factors empower individuals to make informed choices that positively Impact blood sugar levels.

A gestational diabetes-friendly diet focuses on balanced meals and snacks. Choosing complex carbohydrates, lean proteins, and healthy fats helps regulate blood sugar levels. Portion control and mindful eating are essential practices. It's not about deprivation but about making wise food choices that contribute to stable glucose levels.

Physical Activity and Blood Sugar Control

Regular physical activity is beneficial during pregnancy, aiding in blood sugar control. Safe and effective exercises, approved by healthcare providers, contribute to improved insulin sensitivity and overall health. Incorporating physical activity into daily routines helps manage blood sugar levels effectively.

Medication Management

In some cases, medication may be prescribed to manage gestational diabetes. It's crucial to follow healthcare provider instructions regarding medication use. Understanding potential side effects, if any, and discussing any concerns with the healthcare team is essential for effective management.

Stress can impact blood sugar levels, making stress management a crucial aspect of gestational diabetes care. Relaxation techniques, self-care practices, and ensuring sufficient and quality sleep contribute to overall well-being and blood sugar control.

In conclusion, understanding blood sugar levels is fundamental to managing gestational diabetes. By actively engaging in monitoring, adopting a gestational diabetes-friendly lifestyle, and collaborating with healthcare providers, pregnant individuals can navigate this aspect of pregnancy healthily and empower themselves for a positive pregnancy experience.

Day 1

Breakfast: Nutrient-Packed Berry Smoothie Bowl

Lunch: Grilled Chicken and Avocado Salad

Dinner: Baked Lemon Herb Salmon

Day 2

Breakfast: Quinoa Breakfast Porridge with Almond Butter

Lunch: Quinoa and Vegetable Stuffed Peppers

Dinner: Turkey and Vegetable Skillet

Day 3

Breakfast: Egg White Vegetable Omelette

Lunch: Lentil Soup with Gluten-Free Bread

Dinner: Eggplant and Chickpea Stew

Day 4

Breakfast: Gluten-Free Pumpkin Pancakes

Lunch: Zucchini Noodles with Pesto Sauce

Dinner: Cauliflower Crust Pizza

Day 5

Breakfast: Chia Seed Pudding Parfait

Lunch: Grilled Salmon and Quinoa Bowl

Dinner: Stir-Fried Shrimp with Broccoli

Day 6

Breakfast: Vegetable and Feta Breakfast Casserole

Lunch: Turkey and Vegetable Stir-Fry

Dinner: Grilled Chicken and Vegetable Kebabs

Day 7

Breakfast: Sweet Potato and Turkey Sausage Hash

Lunch: Eggplant Lasagna with Gluten-Free Pasta

Dinner: Spaghetti Squash with Turkey Bolognese

Conclusion

As we conclude this exploration into the intricacies of managing gestational diabetes, it's essential to recognize the strength, resilience, and dedication that each mom-to-be brings to this journey. Navigating the waters of pregnancy, especially with the added challenge of gestational diabetes, requires more than just medical insights; it demands courage, patience, and self-compassion.

In the pursuit of understanding blood sugar levels, dietary adjustments, and the various facets of self-care, remember that you are not alone. Gestational diabetes is not just a medical condition; it's an opportunity for empowerment and growth. It's a chance to connect with your body on a profound level, to make mindful choices that nourish both you and your growing baby.

Amidst the glucose meters, dietary plans, and medication considerations, don't forget to celebrate the small victories — the well-managed blood sugar readings, the moments of self-care, and the support received from healthcare providers, loved ones, and, most importantly, yourself. You are crafting a story of resilience, love, and determination.

As you embark on the chapters ahead, know that this journey is uniquely yours, and you are crafting a narrative that goes beyond the parameters of gestational diabetes. It's a story of love, hope, and the extraordinary power within you to nurture life. Embrace the journey, embrace yourself, and embrace the beautiful life you are bringing into the world.

In the tapestry of motherhood, gestational diabetes is just one thread. You are the weaver, the artist, and the storyteller. With each choice you make, each step you take, and each heartbeat shared with your little one, you are creating a masterpiece of love that will last a lifetime.

May this chapter in your life be filled with moments of grace, self-discovery, and the unwavering belief that, through it all, you are enough. Your love, your effort, and your journey are enough. As you continue this beautiful odyssey, may it be adorned with joy, resilience, and the profound sense of accomplishment that comes from nurturing life, one heartbeat at a time.

With love and admiration for the remarkable journey you are undertaking,

Jerry V. Hatcher.

About the author

Jerry V. Hatcher is a culinary virtuoso and the creative mind behind a collection of exquisite cookbooks that transcend the ordinary. With a passion for gastronomy and a flair for culinary artistry, Jerry has crafted a series of cookbooks that take readers on a delectable journey through the world of flavors.

Through his cookbooks, Jerry V. Hatcher combines the finest ingredients with meticulous instructions, ensuring every recipe is a delightful masterpiece waiting to be savored. From tantalizing appetizers to mouthwatering main courses and divine desserts, each page is a celebration of culinary excellence.

With a keen eye for detail, Jerry's cookbooks go beyond the recipes, providing valuable tips, techniques, and personal insights that elevate the cooking experience to new heights. Whether you're a seasoned chef or a culinary enthusiast exploring the kitchen for the first time, Jerry's books cater to all skill levels, fostering confidence and creativity in every home cook.

Each recipe in Jerry V. Hatcher's cookbooks is a reflection of his commitment to authenticity and a passion for diverse cuisines. Drawing inspiration from global flavors and local delicacies, Jerry's culinary creations celebrate the richness of cultures and the joy of sharing food with loved ones. Indulge your passion for cooking and elevate your culinary skills with the culinary masterpieces crafted by Jerry V. Hatcher. Get ready to embark on a gastronomic adventure that will leave you hungry for more, one delicious recipe at a time.

My Little Request

If you have gotten to this point, chances are high you have finished this book.

Thank You for Reading My Book!

I love hearing what you have to say.

I need your input to make the next version of this

book and my future books better.

Please take two minutes now to leave a helpful review on Amazon letting me know what you thought of the book

Thank you so much!

- Jerry V. Hatcher